A narrative of the proceedings relative to the discovery of the longitude at sea; by Mr. John Harrison's time-keeper; subsequent to those published in the year 1763.

John Harrison

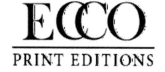

A narrative of the proceedings relative to the discovery of the longitude at sea; by Mr. John Harrison's time-keeper; subsequent to those published in the year 1763.
Harrison, John
ESTCID: T060582
Reproduction from British Library
With a half-title.
London : printed for the author, and sold by Mr. Sandby, 1765.
[4],18p. ; 8°

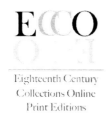

Eighteenth Century
Collections Online
Print Editions

Gale ECCO Print Editions

Relive history with *Eighteenth Century Collections Online*, now available in print for the independent historian and collector. This series includes the most significant English-language and foreign-language works printed in Great Britain during the eighteenth century, and is organized in seven different subject areas including literature and language; medicine, science, and technology; and religion and philosophy. The collection also includes thousands of important works from the Americas.

The eighteenth century has been called "The Age of Enlightenment." It was a period of rapid advance in print culture and publishing, in world exploration, and in the rapid growth of science and technology – all of which had a profound impact on the political and cultural landscape. At the end of the century the American Revolution, French Revolution and Industrial Revolution, perhaps three of the most significant events in modern history, set in motion developments that eventually dominated world political, economic, and social life.

In a groundbreaking effort, Gale initiated a revolution of its own: digitization of epic proportions to preserve these invaluable works in the largest online archive of its kind. Contributions from major world libraries constitute over 175,000 original printed works. Scanned images of the actual pages, rather than transcriptions, recreate the works ***as they first appeared.***

Now for the first time, these high-quality digital scans of original works are available via print-on-demand, making them readily accessible to libraries, students, independent scholars, and readers of all ages.

For our initial release we have created seven robust collections to form one the world's most comprehensive catalogs of 18th century works.

Initial Gale ECCO Print Editions collections include:

> ***History and Geography***
> Rich in titles on English life and social history, this collection spans the world as it was known to eighteenth-century historians and explorers. Titles include a wealth of travel accounts and diaries, histories of nations from throughout the world, and maps and charts of a world that was still being discovered. Students of the War of American Independence will find fascinating accounts from the British side of conflict.

Social Science
Delve into what it was like to live during the eighteenth century by reading the first-hand accounts of everyday people, including city dwellers and farmers, businessmen and bankers, artisans and merchants, artists and their patrons, politicians and their constituents. Original texts make the American, French, and Industrial revolutions vividly contemporary.

Medicine, Science and Technology
Medical theory and practice of the 1700s developed rapidly, as is evidenced by the extensive collection, which includes descriptions of diseases, their conditions, and treatments. Books on science and technology, agriculture, military technology, natural philosophy, even cookbooks, are all contained here.

Literature and Language
Western literary study flows out of eighteenth-century works by Alexander Pope, Daniel Defoe, Henry Fielding, Frances Burney, Denis Diderot, Johann Gottfried Herder, Johann Wolfgang von Goethe, and others. Experience the birth of the modern novel, or compare the development of language using dictionaries and grammar discourses.

Religion and Philosophy
The Age of Enlightenment profoundly enriched religious and philosophical understanding and continues to influence present-day thinking. Works collected here include masterpieces by David Hume, Immanuel Kant, and Jean-Jacques Rousseau, as well as religious sermons and moral debates on the issues of the day, such as the slave trade. The Age of Reason saw conflict between Protestantism and Catholicism transformed into one between faith and logic -- a debate that continues in the twenty-first century.

Law and Reference
This collection reveals the history of English common law and Empire law in a vastly changing world of British expansion. Dominating the legal field is the *Commentaries of the Law of England* by Sir William Blackstone, which first appeared in 1765. Reference works such as almanacs and catalogues continue to educate us by revealing the day-to-day workings of society.

Fine Arts
The eighteenth-century fascination with Greek and Roman antiquity followed the systematic excavation of the ruins at Pompeii and Herculaneum in southern Italy; and after 1750 a neoclassical style dominated all artistic fields. The titles here trace developments in mostly English-language works on painting, sculpture, architecture, music, theater, and other disciplines. Instructional works on musical instruments, catalogs of art objects, comic operas, and more are also included.

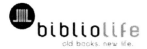

The BiblioLife Network

This project was made possible in part by the BiblioLife Network (BLN), a project aimed at addressing some of the huge challenges facing book preservationists around the world. The BLN includes libraries, library networks, archives, subject matter experts, online communities and library service providers. We believe every book ever published should be available as a high-quality print reproduction; printed on-demand anywhere in the world. This insures the ongoing accessibility of the content and helps generate sustainable revenue for the libraries and organizations that work to preserve these important materials.

The following book is in the "public domain" and represents an authentic reproduction of the text as printed by the original publisher. While we have attempted to accurately maintain the integrity of the original work, there are sometimes problems with the original work or the micro-film from which the books were digitized. This can result in minor errors in reproduction. Possible imperfections include missing and blurred pages, poor pictures, markings and other reproduction issues beyond our control. Because this work is culturally important, we have made it available as part of our commitment to protecting, preserving, and promoting the world's literature.

GUIDE TO FOLD-OUTS MAPS and OVERSIZED IMAGES

The book you are reading was digitized from microfilm captured over the past thirty to forty years. Years after the creation of the original microfilm, the book was converted to digital files and made available in an online database.

In an online database, page images do not need to conform to the size restrictions found in a printed book. When converting these images back into a printed bound book, the page sizes are standardized in ways that maintain the detail of the original. For large images, such as fold-out maps, the original page image is split into two or more pages

Guidelines used to determine how to split the page image follows:

• Some images are split vertically; large images require vertical and horizontal splits.
• For horizontal splits, the content is split left to right.
• For vertical splits, the content is split from top to bottom.
• For both vertical and horizontal splits, the image is processed from top left to bottom right.

A NARRATIVE

OF THE

Proceedings, &c.

Concerning the LONGITUDE.

(Price Sixpence.)

A NARRATIVE

OF THE

PROCEEDINGS

RELATIVE TO

The DISCOVERY of

THE

Longitude at Sea;

BY

Mr. *JOHN HARRISON*'s

TIME-KEEPER;

Subsequent to those published in the Year 1763.

LONDON:

Printed for the AUTHOR, and Sold by Mr. SANDBY, in Fleet-Street.

MDCCLXV.

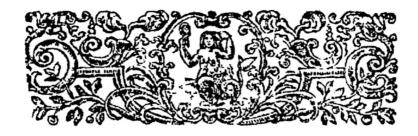

A

NARRATIVE

OF THE

PROCEEDINGS, &c.

N Consequence of the several Matters mentioned in the former Account, a Petition was presented to the Honourable the House of Commons on the Behalf of Mr *John Harrison*, setting forth the material Facts in the Account published in 1763, praying the Assistance of Parliament: which Petition was referred to a Committee, where, (by his Majesty's special Recommendation) the Truth of the Allegations of the said Petition were carefully examined and proved, to the Satisfaction of the Committee: on whose Report an Act was brought into the House, and passed, in which, after reciting

ing 'That the Utility of the Invention of the said *John Harrison* had been proved in a late Voyage to *Jamaica*, under the Directions of the Commissioners of the Longitude,' it was enacted, *That Mr. Harrison should immediately receive the Sum of 5,000 l, Part of the Reward given for the Discovery of the Longitude, on the Terms in the said Act mentioned, viz. on the Discovery of the Principles of his said Instrument, or Watch, for the Discovery of the Longitude, and of the true Manner and Method in which the same is and may be constructed, to Commissioners named in the said Act, and the Residue to be paid so soon as it should appear by future Trial, or Trials, that the said Instrument, or Watch, invented by the said* John Harrison, *should be a proper Method for finding out the Longitude, within the Limits prescribed by the Act of the Twelfth Year of Queen* Anne, *and the said Commissioners of Longitude, or the major Part of them, should certify the same accordingly,* &c. But Difference of Opinion arising amongst the Commissioners appointed by that Act, concerning the Method of carrying this Act into execution, Mr. *Harrison* received no Part of the said 5,000 *l.* so it was thought more for his Benefit, and that of the Publick, that a second Experiment of the Correctness of the Time-keeper should be tried by another Voyage to the *West-Indies*. Barbadoes was fixed on by the Commissioners of Longitude for that Purpose, and accordingly he received the following Instructions.

To

To Mr. *John Harrison,*

ADMIRALTY, *August* 9, 1763.

SIR,

"WHEREAS you have agreed that your Son shall proceed to *Barbadoes,* to make another Trial of your Time keeper, and have desired that such Trial may be made with the Watch only, We have consented thereto, and have applied to the Right Honourable the Lords Commissioners of the Admiralty, for him and your said Machine to be received on board one of his Majesty's Ships, and carried in her to that Island when he shall be ready to proceed, which he informs Us will not be till near *Christmas* next; We desire that in making the said Trial the undermentioned Plan, so far as it relates to you, may be strictly complied with, *viz.*

"FIRST, That your Son does proceed with your said Time-keeper to *Portsmouth,* so soon as it is ready, and it shall be signified to him by our Secretary that a Ship is appointed to receive him on board at that Port; and that, immediately on his Arrival there, three Locks of different Wards be affixed to the Case, in which the said Time-keeper is, in Addition to that which is already to it, and that one of the Keys of those Locks be put in the Possession of *Richard Hughes,* Esq; Commissioner of his Majesty's Navy at that Port, that another be put in Possession of the Captain of the Ship, and that the third be put in Possession of Mr. *John Bradley*, Purser of his Majesty's Ship the *Dorsetshire*, who will be furnished with proper Instruments and Instructions to make Observations of the Sun's equal Altitudes for fixing a Meridian at *Portsmouth*, whereby to compare your Time-keeper; and also to make like Observations for finding the true Time at that Place, on three different Days, at least, previous to your Son's Departure, in the Presence of the said Commissioner *Hughes*, the Captain of the Ship, and your Son; which Observations, together with the Times shewn by your Time-keeper, are to be noted down each Day, and an exact Account thereof, attested by the said Mr. *Bradley*, and the three Persons last-mentioned, to be sent by the same Post, sealed up, to the Secretary of the Admiralty, and they are to compare your Time-keeper with the true Time before your Son proceeds on his Voyage, who is to send an Account of the Rate of the said Time-keeper's Going, sealed up, to the Secretary of the Admiralty, by which you are to abide upon Trial.

"SECONDLY, On your Son's going on shipboard with your said Time-keeper, the First Lieutenant of the Ship is to have the Key from Commissioner *Hughes*, and the Second Lieutenant, or Officer next in Command to the First Lieutenant, is to have that from Mr. *Bradley*, which two Officers with the Captain are

are to be present whenever your Son visits your said Time-keeper on the Voyage.

"THIRDLY, The Reverend Mr. *Nevil Maskelyne*, F. R. S. and Mr. *John Robison*,* (two Persons well skill'd in Astronomy, who will be furnished with proper Instruments) are to go out shortly to *Barbadoes*, in his Majesty's Ship the *Princess Louisa*, to make Observations of the Sun's equal Altitudes for fixing a Meridian there, whereby to compare your Time-keeper, and also to make like Observations on your Son's Arrival, and on two different Days afterwards, at least (and more if it can be done conveniently) in order to find the true Time; which last Observations are to be made in the Presence of the Captain and First Lieutenant of the Ship which carries out your said Time-keeper and your Son, and the said Observations together with the Time shewn by your Time-keeper, are to be noted down each Day, and an exact Account thereof to be sent sealed up, separately, by the first safe Conveyance that offers, to the Secretary of the Admiralty, attested by the said Mr. *Maskelyne*, Mr. *Robison*, and the four other Persons last-mentioned, in whose Presence the Observations are to be made; and it is to be understood, that if it should so happen, by the Interruption of

* Mr. *Robison* not being able to go the Voyage, Mr. *Charles Green*, Assistant to the Royal Astronomer at *Greenwich*, was ordered by the Commissioners to go in his Stead.

Clouds,

Clouds, that only one correspondent equal Altitude can be had, on all or any of the Days on which they are to make the Observations, that then such one correspondent equal Altitude shall be a sufficient Observation for the Day on which the same shall be taken.

"FOURTHLY, The abovementioned Mr. *Maskelyne* and Mr. *Robison* are to make as many and as accurate Observations as possible of the Eclipses of *Jupiter's* first Satellite, when the same shall be visible at *Barbadoes*, as well of its Immersions as Emersions, and also of as many Occultations of the fixt Stars and Planets as may be visible at that Island, and correspondent Observations will be made thereof at *Portsmouth*, and at the Royal Observatory at *Greenwich*, by Instruments exactly similar to those which the said Mr. *Maskelyne* and Mr. *Robison* will be furnished with in order to determine the Difference of the Meridians of that Island and *Portsmouth*.

We heartily wish you Success in this Undertaking, and are, Sir, &c."

On the 4th of *February* 1764, Mr. *William Harrison* received the following Letter from Mr. *Stephens*;

Admiralty-Office, *Feb.* 4, 1764.

SIR,

"CApt. *Lindsay* of his Majesty's Ship *Tartar*, now at *Deptford*, being directed to proceed as soon as possible to *Spithead*, where

where he will receive Orders for proceeding to the *West-Indies*, after having assisted at the Observations which are to be made at *Portsmouth* for the Trial of your Father's Time-keeper; and he being also directed to receive you, and Mr. *Thomas Wyatt*, your Companion, and the said Time-keeper, with your Baggage, on board the said Ship, and give you a Passage to *Barbadoes*, in Order for your making a second Trial of your Father's said Time-keeper. I am to acquaint you therewith, and am, Sir,

Your very humble Servant,
PHILIP STEPHENS."

The *Tartar* sailed from *Spithead* the 28th of *March*, and met with hard and contrary Gales; especially in the *Bay of Biscay*. *April* the 19th they made the Island of *Porto Santo*, North East of the *Madeiras*, as set forth in the following Certificate of Sir *John Lindsay*.

Madeira, April 19, 1764.
" I do hereby certify, that Yesterday at
" Four o'Clock in the Afternoon, Mr. *Willi-*
" *am Harrison* took two Altitudes of the Sun
" to ascertain the Difference of Longitude
" given by the Time-keeper from *Portf-*
" *mouth*; according to which Observations
" he declared to me, we were at that Time
" 43 Miles to the Eastward of *Porto Santo*. I
" then steered a direct Course for it, and at
" One o'Clock this Morning we saw the
" Island,

" Island, which exactly agreed with the
" Distance mentioned above.
  " Given under my Hand on board his
  " Majesty's Ship the *Tarta*.
                    JOHN LINDSAY."

They arrived at *Barbadoes* Ma the 13th, Mr. *Harrison* all along in the Voyage declaring how far he was distant from that Island, according to the best settled Longitude thereof. The Day before they made it, he declared the Distance: and Sir *John* sailed in Consequence of this Declaration, till Eleven at Night, which proving dark he thought proper to lay by. Mr. *Harrison* then declaring they were no more than eight or nine Miles from the Land, which accordingly at Day Break they saw from that Distance.

At a Meeting of the Commissioners appointed by Act of Parliament for the Discovery of the Longitude, &c. held at the Admiralty on *Tuesday* the 18th of *September*, 1764, Mr. *Stephens* laid before the Board the Letter which he had received, as Secretary of the Admiralty, from Mr. *Harrison*, containing his Declaration of the Rate of the Going of his Time-keeper, and also the several Letters which he had received from Mr. *Bradley*, Mr. *Maskelyne*, and Mr. *Green*, containing the Observations that have been made by them in Obedience to the Instructions which had been given them: Which being read, the Board came to the following Resolutions;
  " That

" That the said Observations be reduced to apparent Time:

That the Longitude be deduced from corresponding Observations, if any; but if there be no corresponding Observations, that Mr. *Waggentine*'s last Tables of *Jupiter*'s Satellites, corrected by Observations, be used for making the Comparisons, but at no greater Distance of Time from one another, than six Revolutions of the first Satellite, and that the Comparisons be marked down, and the Results severally flowing therefrom.

That the Longitude be also deduced from the correspondent Observations of Occultations of fixt Stars and Planets, if there be any correspondent Observations, either at the Royal Observatory at *Greenwich*, or among the Observations taken by Mr. *Bradley* at *Portsmouth*.

That Mr. *Hornsby* and Mr. *Green* do extract the Observations of the first Satellite of *Jupiter*, and the Occultations of the fixt Stars and Planets, from the 15th of *November* 1763, to the 3d of *March* 1764, from the Observation Book at *Greenwich*; and certify that the Observations are faithfully copied, and that Mr. *Harrison*'s Son be present at the extracting the said Observations, and sign the Certificate, if he chuses it.

Resolved,

That the said Observations be referred to three Gentlemen of Skill, to make the Calculations mentioned in the aforesaid Resolutions; and that Mr. *Harrison* be at Liberty to name three Persons also, for the same Purpose.

Captain *John Campbell*, and Doctor *Bevis*, were named, by some Members of the Board, as very proper Persons to make those Calculations; and being called in, and severally asked if it would be agreeable to them to undertake the Trouble of making the said Calculations; they answered in the Affirmative, and then withdrew.

Mr. *Shepherd*, one of the Members of the Board, mentioned Mr. *George Witchell*, as a proper Person to be added to the two Gentlemen above-named, and said he would answer for his undertaking it; and the Board approved of Mr. *Witchell*.

Resolved,

That Copies of Mr. *Harrison*'s Declaration of the Rate of the Going of his Time-keeper before he left *Portsmouth*, together with Copies of the Observations that have been transmitted to the Secretary of the Admiralty from Mr. *Bradley*, Mr. *Maskelyne*, and Mr. *Green*; and also the Observations collated with the Observation Book at *Greenwich*, be sent to Captain *Campbell*, Doctor *Bevis*, and Mr. *Witchell*; respectively, after they shall have been examined and attested by Mr. *Harrison*, or his Son; in order to their making the said Calculations; and that they be requested to return their Calculations by the last Day of *October*, if it suits with their Conveniency.

After these Resolutions of the Commissioners of Longitude, Mr. *John Harrison* presented to them the following Memorial, dated the 19th *January*, 1765.

To the Right Honourable, and Honourable, the Commissioners constituted for the Discovery of the Longitude at Sea; and for examining and judging of all Proposals, Experiments, and Improvements, relating to the same.

The MEMORIAL *of* JOHN HARRISON, *of* Red Lyon Square, *in the Parish of Saint* George the Martyr, Queen-Square, London;

Humbly sheweth,

" THAT, whereas by an Act made in the 12th Year of her late Majesty Queen *Anne*, intitled, An Act for providing a public Reward for such Person or Persons as shall discover the Longitude at Sea, it is, amongst other Things, enacted

" That after Experiments made of any
" Proposal, or Proposals, for the Discovery
" of the said Longitude, the Commissioners
" appointed by the said Act (or the major
" Part of them) shall declare and determine
" how far the same is found practicable, and
" to what Degree of Exactness.

" That for a due Encouragement to any
" such Person or Persons as shall discover a
" proper Method for finding the said Lon-
" gitude, it is enacted, that the first Author,

" or

" or Authors, Difcoverer, or Difcoverers, of
" any fuch Method, his or their Executors,
" Adminiftrators, or Affigns, fhall be entitled
" to, and have, fuch Rewards or Sum, as is
" therein after mentioned; that is to fay, a
" Reward of 10,000 *l.* if it determines the
" faid Longitude to one Degree of a great
" Circle, or *Sixty* geographical Miles, to
" 15,000 *l.* if it determines the fame to two
" Thirds of that Diftance, and to 20,000 *l.*
" if it determines the fame to one Half of
" that Diftance; one Moiety, or half
" Part to be paid when the faid Commiffio-
" ners, or the major Part of them, do agree
" that any fuch Method extends to the Secu-
" rity of Ships within *Eighty* geographical
" Miles of the Shores which are Places of
" the greateft Danger, and the other Moiety
" or half Part when a Ship, by the Appoint-
" ment of the faid Commiffioners, or the
" Majority of them, fhall thereby actually
" fail over the Ocean, from *Great Britain*, to
" any fuch Port in the *Weft Indies*, as thofe
" Commiffioners, or the major Part of them,
" fhall choofe or nominate for the Experi-
" ment, without lofeing their Longitude be-
" yond the Limits before-mentioned."

By the faid Act it is further enacted, "That
" as foon as fuch Method for the Difcovery
" of the faid Longitude fhall have been tried
" and found practicable and ufeful at Sea,
" within any of the Degrees aforefaid, that
" the faid Commiffioners, or the major Part
" of them, fhall certify the fame according-
" ly.

"ly, under their Hands and Seals, to the
"Commissioners of the Navy for the Time
"being; together with the Person or Persons
"names, who are the Authors of such Pro-
"posals: and upon such Certificate, the said
"Commissioners are thereby authorised and
"required to make out a Bill or Bills for the
"respective Sum, or Sums, of Money to
"which the Author, or Authors, of such
"Proposals, their Executors, Administrators
"or Assigns, shall be Entitled, by virtue of
"this Act."

And Whereas a method (invented by your Memorialist) for the Discovery of the Longitude hath been tried by Experiments made according to the Appointment of your Honourable Board; by which Method a Ship hath sailed over the Ocean from *Great-Britain* to the *West-Indies*, (according to the Instructions of your Honourable Board of the 9th of *August* 1763) to wit, His Majesty's Ship *Tartar*, under the Command of Sir *John Lindsay*, from *Portsmouth* to the Island of *Barbadoes*, without losing the Longitude beyond the nearest Limits mentioned in the said Act, as appears by the several Testimonials and Certificates relative to the said Experiments, which have been transmitted to your Honourable Board, in Obedience to your Orders and Instructions, to which Orders and Instructions your Memorialist hath in all things conformed.

" And whereas your Memorialist, by Order of your Honourable Board hath received 2,500 *l.* in Part of the Money directed by the said *Act* to be paid to the Author of such Discovery.

Your Memorialist therefore humbly prays; that your Honourable Board will be pleased to grant him such Certificate as is directed by the above recited Act.

And your Memorialist as in Duty bound shall ever pray,
Jan. 19 1765.   JOHN HARRISON.

In Answer to this Memorial, Mr. *Harrison* received the following Resolutions.

At a Meeting of the Commissioners appointed by Act of Parliament for the Discovery of the Longitude at Sea, &c. which was held at the Admiralty on *Saturday* the 9th of *February*, 1765.

" Mr. *Harrison*'s Memorial, which was laid before the last Board, was again read; and the Commissioners present, having taken into Consideration the Difference of Longitude

tude between *Portsmouth* in *Great-Britain*, and *Bridge-Town* in his Majesty's Island of *Barbadoes*, resulting from a Mean of corresponding astronomical Observations made at both Places, agreeable to the Resolution of this Board of the 4th and 9th of *August* 1763, and to the Instructions given in Consequence thereof, and having compared the said Difference with the Difference of Longitude between the said Places, given by Mr. *John Harrison*'s Time-keeper, they are unanimously of Opinion, that the said Time-keeper has kept its Time with sufficient Exactness, and without loseing its Longitude in the Voyage from *Portsmouth* to *Barbadoes*, beyond the nearest Limit required by the Act of the 12th of Queen *Anne*, but even considerably within the same; but, in regard the said Mr. *John Harrison* hath not yet made a Discovery of the Principles upon which his said Time-keeper is constructed, nor of the Method of carrying those Principles into Execution, by Means whereof other such Time-keepers might be framed, of sufficient Correctness to find the Longitude at Sea, within the Limits by the said Act required, whereby the said Invention might be adjudged practicable and useful in Terms of the said Act, and agreeable to the true Intent and Meaning thereof, the Commissioners do not therefore think themselves authorised to grant any Certificate to the said Mr. *John Harrison*, until he shall have made a full and clear Discovery of the said Principles and Method, and

the

the same shall have been found practicable and useful to their Satisfaction. But they are notwithstanding of Opinion, that Application should be made to Parliament for Leave to pay the said Mr. *John Harrison*, upon his producing his Time-keeper to certain Persons to be named by this Board, and discovering to them the Principles and Manner of making the same, so much Money as will make up the Sums already advanced to him 10,000 *l.* exclusive of what he has received on Account of improving his said Time-keeper; and moreover to pay him the Remainder of the Reward of 20,000 *l.* on Proof being made to the Satisfaction of this Board, that his Method will be of common and general Utility in finding the Longitude at Sea, within the nearest Limits required by the abovementioned Act of the 12th of Queen *Anne*.

" Mr. *Harrison*'s Son, who was attending, was called in, and acquainted with these Resolutions, a Copy of which he desired might be sent to his Father, and then withdrew.
Resolved,
That a Copy of the same be sent to Mr. *John Harrison* accordingly, in Answer to his before-mentioned Memorial."

Now as by the last Act of Parliament it appears that the Utility of Mr. *Harrison*'s Timekeeper has been fully proved; and also by the Reso-

Resolutions of the Honourable Commissioners of the 9th of this Instant *February*, that the said Time-keeper has kept its Time with sufficient Exactness, and without loseing its Longitude beyond the nearest Limits required by the Act of the 12th of Queen *Anne*, but even considerably within the same: Mr. *Harrison* humbly hopes, that if any Application should be made to Parliament, relative to his Invention; that he shall not, thereby, be deprived of receiving the Residue of the 20000*l.* to which he apprehends himself legally intitled, in Consequence of the Success of his Invention, by Virtue of the Acts of Parliament before-mentioned.

Mr. *John Harrison*, in order to satisfy any Doubts or Scruples, that can possibly arise; and to the End that his Invention may not be lost to the Public, by the Accident of his, or his Son's Death; hath offered, and is willing, to deliver to the Honourable the Commissioners of the Longitude, or to the Lords of Admiralty, his Time-keeper: by which any other skilful Workman may be enabled to make other Time-keepers on the same Principles. And, for a farther Satisfaction, he is willing to deposit, in the Hands of the Lords of the Admiralty, correct Drawings upon Oath, with Explanations of such Drawings; and also of the Principles on which the same is constructed.

Mr. *Harrison* should hope, that what is above proposed, will be a sufficient Proof of his sincere Desire that the Public, may, so soon as possible, reap the Benefit of his Invention: yet, for the farther Satisfaction of the Public, he is willing to engage his Son, immediately on his receiving the Reward given by the Legislature, to employ a sufficient Number of Hands, so as with all possible Speed to furnish his Majesty's Navy, the Merchants and Navigators of this Kingdom, with such Number of Time-keepers, of equal Goodness with that already made, and in two Voyages incontestably proved, at such reasonable Rates, as the Nature of the Undertaking will admit: not doubting but the Public will consider the Charge attending the Outset of the Undertaking.

Mr. *Harrison* hopes these Proposals will be thought satisfactory to the Public; without subjecting him to those Delays, and Inconveniences, as might probably attend the Methods proposed by the Honourable the Commissioners of the Longitude; as he is already very infirm, and far advanced in Years, above 40 whereof have been entirely taken up in this Service alone. Moreover if the Method proposed by Mr. *Harrison* be approved of, the Public will be secured from any Imposition by Counterfeits. Mr. *Harrison* likewise would not be deprived of the Rewards he may receive from foreign Nations to whom he may communicate his Discovery.

F I N I S.

The following is a Copy of Mr William Harrison's declaration of the rate of the going of his Time-keeper which according to his Instructions he was to send to Mr Stephens before he left Portsmouth.

To the Right Honourable and Honourable the Commissioners of Longitude.

My Lords and Gentlemen

In obedience to your Instructions dated the 9th of August 1763 I humbly Certify that I do expect the rate of the going of the Time-keeper will be as followeth viz.

When the Thermometer is at 42, it will gain 3 seconds in every 24 Hours.

Wm

When the Thermometer is at 52, it will gain 2 Seconds in every 24 Hours.

When the Thermometer is at 62, it will gain 1 Second in every 24 Hours.

When the Thermometer is at 72, it will neither gain nor lose.

When the Thermometer is at 82, it will lose 1 Second in every 24 Hours.

Since my last Voyage we have made some improvement in the Time keeper, in consequence of which the Provision to counter-balance the effects of Heat and Cold has been made anew, and for the want of a little more time we could not get it quite adjusted for which

reason the above allowances are
necessary.

This is its present state, and
as the inequalities are so small, it
will abide by the rate of its gaining
on a mean one second a Day for
the Voyage.

I would not be understood that
it will always require so long time
to bring those Machines to perfection
for it is well known to be much harder
to beat out a new Road than it is to
follow that Road when made.

During the Time of this experiment the mean hight of the Thermometer shall be each day carefully
noted down and Certified which I
will lay before the Board at my return.

I am Your most Obedient
and most humble Serv.t
William Harrison

Portsmouth
Mar 26 1764

In the following Account the first Column is the day of the Month, the second is the height of the Thermometer, the third how much the Time-keeper was fast by equal Altitudes, the fourth how much it should be fast when allowance is made for the different heights of the Thermometer; and the fifth is supposing it to gain one second a Day from Portsmouth to Barbadoes.

At Portsmouth

1764		h ,	h , ,	h ,
Feby				
29	42	0 4 31.5	0 4 31.5	
March			+3	
1	40	— —	0 4 34.5	
			3.2	
2	42	— —	0 4 37.7	
			3	
3	43	— —	0 4 40.7	
			2.9	
4	44	— —	0 4 43.6	

March

4	44	–	–	–	0	4	43 6
							2 8
5	47	–	–	–	0	4	46 4
							2 5
6	46	–	–	–	0	4	48 9
							2 6
7	46	0	4	51 2	0	4	51 5
							2 6
8	47	–	–	–	0	4	54 1
							2 5
9	48	–	–	–	0	4	56 6
							2 4
10	48	–	–	–	0	4	59 0
							2 4
11	50	–	–	–	0	5	1 4
							2 2
12	52	–	–	–	0	5	3 6
							2 –
13	54	–	–	–	0	5	5 6
							1 8
14	53	0	5	13 7	0	5	7 4
							1 2
15	55	–	–	–	0	5	9 8
							1 2
16	52	–	–	–	0	5	11 0
							2 –
17	56	–	–	–	0	5	13 0
							1 6
18	52	–	–	–	0	5	14 6
							2 –
19	55	–	–	–	0	5	16 6
							1 7
20	51	–	–	–	0	5	18 3

March
20	51	-	-	-	0.5	18.3	
						2.1	
21	52	0.5.2b5			0.5	20.4	0 5 26
						2	
22	51	-	-	-	0 5	22.4	0 5 27
						2.1	
23	53	-	-	-	0 5	24.5	0 5 28
						1.9	
24	52	-	-	-	0 5	26.4	0 5 29
						2	
25	51	-	-	-	0 5	28.4	0 5 30
						1.5	
26	54	-	-	-	0.5	29.9	0 5 31
						1.8	
27	50	-	-	-	0 5	31.7	0 5 32
						2.2	

At Sea

28	49	-	-	-	0 5	33.9	0 5 33
						2.3	
29	51	-	-	-	0 5	36.2	0.5 34
						2.1	
30	53	-	-	-	0 5	38.3	0 5 35
						1.9	
31	55	-	-	-	0 5	40.2	0 5 36
						1.7	

April
1	53	-	-	-	0 5	41.9	0.5 37
						1.9	
2	54	-	-	-	0 5	43.8	0 5 38
						1.8	
3	55	-	-	-	0.5	45.6	0 5 39
						1.7	
4	56	-	-	-	0.5	47.3	0 5 40

April

4	56	-	-	-	0	5	47 3	0 5 40
							1 6	
5	56	-	-	-	0	5	48 9	0 5 41
							1 6	
6	53	-	-	-	0	5	50 5	0 5 42
							1 9	
7	53	-	-	-	0	5	52 4	0 5 43
							1 9	
8	53	-	-	-	0	5	54 3	0 5 44
							1 9	
9	53	-	-	-	0	5	56 2	0 5 45
							1 9	
10	52	-	-	-	0	5	58 1	0 5 46
							2 0	
11	53	-	-	-	0	6	0 1	0 5 47
							1 9	
12	58	-	-	-	0	6	2 0	0 5 48
							1 4	
13	56	-	-	-	0	6	3 4	0 5 49
							1 6	
14	58	-	-	-	0	6	5 0	0 5 50
							1 4	
15	61	-	-	-	0	6	6 4	0 5 51
							1 1	
16	63	-	-	-	0	6	7 5	0 5 52
							9	
17	65	-	-	-	0	6	8 4	0 5 53
							7	
18	66	-	-	-	0	6	9 1	0 5 54
							6	
19	67	-	-	-	0	6	9 7	0 5 55
							5	
20	70	-	-	-	0	6	10 2	0 5 56

April									
20	70	-	-	-	-	0	6	10 2	0 5 56
								2	
21	69	-	-	-	-	0	6	10 4	0 5 57
								·3	
22	70	-	-	-	-	0	6	10 7	0 5 58
								·2	
23	69	-	-	-	-	0	6	10 9	0 5 59
								3	
24	66	-	-	-	-	0	6	11 2	0 6 0
								·6	
25	68	-	-	-	-	0	6	11 8	0 6 1
								4	
26	69	-	-	-	-	0	6.	12 2	0 6.2
								3	
27	70	-	-	-	-	0	6	12 5	0 6.3
								2	
28	71	-	-	-	-	0	6	12 7	0 6 4
								1	
29	73	-	-	-	-	0	6	12 8	0.6 5
								−1	
30	71	-	-	-	-	0	6	12 7	0.6.6
								+1	
May									
1	73	-	-	-	-	0	6	12 8	0 6 7
								−1	
2	74	-	-	-	-	0	6	12 7	0 6 8
								−2	
3	74	-	-	-	-	0	6	12 5	0 6 9
								−2	
4	75	-	-	-	-	0	6.	12 3	0 6 10
								−3	
5	77	-	-	-	-	0	6.	12 0	0 6 11
								−5	
6	79	-	-	-	-	0	6	11 5	0.6.12

May

6	79	-	-	-	o	b	11.5	0 b	12
							−7		
7	79	-	-	-	o	b	10.8	0 b	13
							7		
8	79	-	-	-	o	b	10.1	0 b	14
							1		
9	80	-	-	-	o	b	9.4	0 b	15
							8		
10	81	-	-	-	o	b	8.6	0 b	16
							.9		
11	82	-	-	-	0.	b	7.5	0 b	17
							1		
12	82	-	-	-	o	b	6.5	0. b	18
							1		
13	82	-	-	-	o	b	5.5	o b	19
							1		

Barbadoes

14	85	4.1	13.5	0	b	4.5	0.b	20
						1.3		
15	84	4.1	11.	0.b	3.2	0 b	21
						1.2		
16	85	4.1.8	2 0.b	2.0	0 b	22
						1.3		
17	84	4.1	7	0 b.	0.7	0.b	23

Barbadoes

May the 14th Timekeeper fast of
Barbadoes time by Equal Alti-
tude _ _ _ _ _ _ _ _ _ _ _ _ _ 4. 1 15 s^{h}

Supposing the time keeper
to gain one Second a Day
for the voyage it will be fast
of Portsmouth time _ _ _ 0 6 20

difference _ _ _ _ _ _ _ _ _ _ 3 54 35 s

which is Equal to _ _ _ _ _ _ 58. 44°

Difference of Longitude
by Jupiters Satellite _ _ 58 34 ½

difference _ _ _ _ 0 9 ½

Lightning Source UK Ltd.
Milton Keynes UK
16 February 2011
167628UK00005B/95/P